Never Accept a Lift
from Strangers

How to Choose the Best Plastic Surgeon
for your Cosmetic Breast Surgery

Dear Laura,

Enjoy the book!

Jonathan

Jonathan Staiano
Staiano Plastic Surgery

ISBN-13: 978-1535038386

Published by
10-10-10 Publishing
Markham, Ontario
CANADA

Contents

FOREWORD

If you are considering cosmetic surgery this book is a must read. It is frightening to think that plastic surgery is being performed by non-plastic surgeons both in the UK and in the USA. Jonathan Staiano has lifted the lid on something that you would never be aware of.

Cosmetic surgery is an everyday procedure these days and there is an element of trust in your doctor. You cannot assume that your doctor has been trained to perform your procedure, the burden is on you to check.

Never Accept a Lift from Strangers clearly explains what you should look for in your surgeon and gives you a balanced overview of the cosmetic surgery industry. Jonathan has a great way of writing and I found this book to be easy to read and a fascinating insight into the higher levels of surgical training. If you or someone you know are thinking of having surgery, read this book first.

Do not speak to a plastic surgeon until you have read this book.

Raymond Aaron
New York Times Bestselling Author

INTRODUCTION

Who is this book for?

This book is for anyone considering cosmetic surgery, or any other type of surgery for that matter - although in other fields of surgery, surgeons tend to stick within their scope of practice and there is not as much hype and marketing as there is with cosmetic surgery.

It is also for anyone who has a friend or relative who may be considering surgery, as you will be able to help with the research process and provide support and counsel during what can be a confusing and emotional time.

Finally, it is for anyone who is interested in the medical profession and is looking for an insight into what it takes to become a Specialist Consultant Surgeon. Surgical training in the UK, and Plastic Surgery in particular, is a competitive and lengthy affair and can take around 15-20 years to complete. I will break down what is involved in this time and explain the differences between the different surgical specialities. The medical profession has for a long time had the reputation of being a closed group with a paternalistic attitude. There was a time when patients would be grateful to be seen by a doctor and would accept their advice and recommendations without question. However, times have changed.

Everyone is an expert these days

We are now in a world where the knowledge acquired through years of study and training can be accessed in the fraction of a second by anyone with a computer and an internet connection. We are no longer dependant on experts or professionals for information, because the information is freely available to us all.

However, we do need professionals with experience who can interpret the facts and we need experts with technical ability to perform procedures for us.

In this book I will help you to understand the information that is out there. All doctors should provide details about their training, but unfortunately it is not always clear and easy to find. I will explain what all the letters mean after a doctor's name and what it means to be a member of the various surgical societies and colleges. I will go through what it takes to become a specialist in a particular field and uncover the reality that many doctors in the cosmetic surgery industry have no formal specialist training at all.

About me

My name is Jonathan Staiano and I am a Consultant Plastic Surgeon with a special interest in cosmetic breast surgery. In this book I will explain what this means and why I have written about it.

Over the years, I have become increasingly aware of the number of operations performed by people who may not have the best qualifications to be performing the procedure. What I aim to do with this book is to clearly and concisely explain what is involved in surgical training and to give you the ability to tell whether a surgeon has the appropriate training to be performing your procedure.

Despite the complexity of what a surgeon does, the cosmetic surgery industry is largely unregulated and the onus is on you as a patient to choose your surgeon wisely. I hope that this book will give you the information that you need to let you make an informed decision about who you allow to operate on you. There are many excellent surgeons out there who perform outstanding work and provide excellent care; I hope that I can help you to find one of them.

"I will uncover the reality that many doctors in the cosmetic surgery industry have no formal specialist training at all"

WHAT MAKES A SPECIALIST?

What do all the qualifications mean?

Training is crucial in surgery and it is important to be aware of what all the qualifications mean. Some doctors may have a line of initials after their name and look very impressive, while others may prefer to keep things simple and just use their highest qualification. This means that you cannot always tell by the number of letters after a doctor's name, how qualified they are.

It helps to have an idea of what the important qualifications are, then you can just look for these.

Basic qualifications for all doctors

All doctors will be registered with the General Medical Council (GMC). This is a basic requirement and is achieved after one year of practising medicine (following six years of medical training at University). All doctors are encouraged to share their GMC number and you can check whether your doctor is registered with the GMC on their website (www.gmc-uk.org) using the GMC number or the doctor's name. When a doctor qualifies in medicine they receive the letters after their name of MB BS, or MB ChB (this stands for Bachelor of Medicine and Bachelor of Surgery – Surgery is Chirugie in Latin – hence the Ch). If your surgeon is not registered with the GMC, then they will not be a qualified doctor and so they may be a dentist, a nurse, or have other paramedical qualifications – but this would be a cause for some concern and you should certainly do further research in to their qualifications and their suitability to perform your procedure.

Many doctors will do another degree, either before or during their medical degree and so they may also have BSc or BA after their name (this stands for Bachelor of Science or Bachelor of Arts). These qualifications show that your doctor may be more academic, but they are not really necessary when it comes to choosing a surgeon.

Most plastic surgeons go on to do higher degrees which involve a period of research and which take on average, an extra 1, 2 or 3 years and will lead to the degrees of MSc, MD or PhD, respectively (these letters stand for Master of Science, Doctor of Medicine and Doctor of Philosophy). Again, these qualifications are impressive because the doctor has done a period of research, but they are not essential when deciding on a surgeon.

Basic training for surgeons – MRCS and FRCS

If a doctor wishes to pursue a career in surgery, they will need to enter a basic surgical training scheme which involves 3-5 years of surgical training across the surgical specialities and then they will be eligible to take an exam at the Royal College of Surgeons to gain membership of the college. Until the doctor has passed this exam, they will not be able to progress on to advanced surgical training and it can take many years to achieve this goal. Being a member or fellow of the Royal College of Surgeons allows you to use the letters MRCS or FRCS after your name (this is the same basic surgical qualification but in 2007 it was changed from a fellowship to a membership). It also allows a doctor to be called Mr - a reference back to the days when surgeons were barbers.

Having the letters MRCS or FRCS and being a member or a fellow of the Royal College of Surgeons may sound like an impressive qualification, but it does not mean that your surgeon is fully trained in a surgical speciality. It only means that your surgeon has reached a basic level of surgical training and is now eligible to undertake advanced training with the view to becoming a specialist.

Advanced training for surgeons – FRCS(Plast)

The big bottleneck in surgical training is between basic and advanced surgical training programs. There are more doctors trying to get on to an advanced training program, than there are programs available. Plastic surgery is one of the longest and most sought after training programs. There are only a small number of places on these schemes because plastic surgery is only performed in major teaching hospitals, so the number of training programs is limited. Most surgical specialities, such as general surgery or orthopaedics are present in all hospitals and there are a lot more of these training places available. This means that some doctors can wait a long time to get on to a training scheme in plastic surgery and many will either not be able to get on to the training program of their choice and have to choose a different speciality or will not be able to progress with advanced training at all.

Once on an advanced training scheme, the surgeon will work in an NHS hospital and will have the job title of Specialist Registrar (SpR) and will undergo six years of specialist training with regular assessments under the supervision of a Consultant. At the end of this training, there is another exam to pass which leads to the award of the FRCS(Plast) qualification, which is the highest qualification that a plastic surgeon can achieve and is a test of whether the surgeon is able to operate independently without supervision.

The FRCS(Plast) qualification after a surgeon's name may look similar to FRCS (or MRCS) but those extra letters in brackets, which signify the speciality in which the surgeon is trained, make a world of difference. A surgeon with FRCS(Plast) after their name is a fully trained plastic surgeon who will have been tested and examined by his peers and has been deemed safe to look after and treat patients autonomously. They can now go on and apply for a Consultant post in the NHS and to have patients who are under their care, who they are responsible for.

However, in the private sector, a surgeon does not have to have this qualification in order to start seeing and treating patients. There is nothing to stop a doctor from setting up a practice in the private sector, even though they would not be able to look after patients in the NHS, unless they were being supervised by a Consultant.

There is no law against it

There is no legislation around who can perform an operation. Many people are operated upon by surgeons who are not fully trained in a speciality and so will only have the basic surgical qualification of FRCS or MRCS. In fact many people are operated upon by doctors who have no formal surgical training at all and so will not even have these letters after their name. This may be acceptable in some areas, such as removal of a mole by a dermatologist, but when it comes to more invasive surgery, then some form of formal surgical training would be advisable.

Jonathan Staiano

CASE STUDY

Footballer's wife dies following liposuction
performed by a GP

Colin Hendry's wife had abdominal liposuction in 2002, suffered multiple perforations of her bowel and had a prolonged post-operative course in intensive care. Sadly, she finally died from her injuries in 2009.

Colin Hendry was a premiership footballer and was the captain of the Scottish National team. He would have wanted the best care and expertise for his wife's surgery yet the surgeon who performed his wife's surgery was a general practitioner from Poland who had no surgical qualification.

There are an increasing number of commercial clinics that offer cosmetic surgery and they tend not to put the surgeon front and centre. They may have a glossy façade and have smooth-talking salespeople and it is easy to be impressed by the sales pitch. However, it is important to remember that cosmetic surgery is not the same as buying a car or having your nails done. It is a medical procedure and it needs to be performed by a qualified medical practitioner. Unfortunately, there is no law against any doctor performing any procedure, even if they have not been trained in it, so the onus is on you as a patient to make sure that your surgeon has the appropriate

6

qualifications (in fact you can start by making sure that they are actually a surgeon, as the doctor in this case had no surgical qualifications).

It is not necessary for your surgeon to be a plastic surgeon, as there are other types of specialists who perform cosmetic surgery; however, you should make sure that you know whether your surgeon has undergone specialist training, and if so, in what. Plastic surgery encompasses all aspects of cosmetic surgery, but there are some specialities that overlap with plastic surgery. ENT (Ear, Nose and Throat) surgeons can be experts in rhinoplasty (nose job) and Ophthalmic (Eye) surgeons can perform eye lifts (blepharoplasty). The case above shows that a doctor does not need to have any formal surgical training to perform surgery and there are many doctors out there who are not surgeons, but are performing surgery. This in itself may not be as shocking as it sounds, as long as you are aware of your doctor's qualifications.

Many dermatologists perform minor skin surgery and may have a wealth of experience in this despite having no formal surgical training. Similarly, General Practitioners will often branch out in to performing cosmetic treatments, which can range from non-surgical procedures such as wrinkle relaxing injections and fillers through to more invasive treatments such as some forms of liposuction and face lifting. They may have many happy patients and you may feel comfortable and safe having them operate on you. The important thing is that you are aware of their level of training so that you can make an informed decision.

"Your surgeon does not need to be a Plastic Surgeon to be trained in Cosmetic Surgery, but you should be aware of what speciality training they have had (if any)"

NOTES

NOTES

WHAT IS A BREAST SURGEON?

What makes a breast surgeon?

There are two types of surgeon who perform breast surgery - plastic surgeons and general surgeons. Both are specialists in their field (even though general surgeons sound like they do everything, they are actually quite specialised) and both should be on the specialist register with the GMC for their chosen speciality. The training is very different and the scope of practice varies between these two types of surgeon.

General surgery training

General surgery, while it sounds as if it is all-encompassing, is actually a speciality in itself. All surgeons need to do some general surgery training before specialising and some choose to specialise in general surgery itself. General surgery training involves surgery of the bowels and the glands (such as thyroid and breast). Aesthetics plays no role. Towards the end of general surgery training, surgeons will be encouraged to sub-specialise, and breast surgery is one of the fields they might choose. The work involves breast cancer diagnosis and management, including removing breast lumps and mastectomy. Some general surgeons will go on to learn to perform breast reconstruction. This group are known as oncoplastic breast surgeons and they will spend one or two years learning about breast reconstruction, although not all oncoplastic surgeons will have been trained by a plastic surgeon.

Plastic surgery training

Plastic surgery training revolves around soft tissue handling and reconstruction. Restoration of function as well as aesthetics plays a key role in all areas of plastic surgery. Cosmetic surgery is not a speciality in itself, but towards the end of plastic surgery training some surgeons will sub-specialise in breast surgery, which will mainly be breast reconstruction after cancer (see chapter 'what is a plastic surgeon'). Plastic surgeons who specialise in the breast, tend to focus on reconstruction following mastectomy, rather than doing the mastectomy itself, and balancing surgery to make the opposite normal breast look like the reconstructed breast. The priority for the plastic surgeon is usually to ensure a good form and symmetry of the breast whereas the general surgeon's priority is to ensure all of the cancer is removed.

The plastic surgeon does not focus on the diagnosis and treatment of breast cancer as this is done by the general breast surgeon. You can tell the difference between a general breast surgeon and a plastic breast surgeon by looking on the GMC website where they will be listed as being on the specialist register for either general surgery or plastic surgery (assuming they are on the specialist register). Alternatively, if you look at the letters after their name, a general breast surgeon will have FRCS(Gen) whereas a plastic breast surgeon will have FRCS(Plast).

CASE STUDY

'If all that you have is a hammer, everything looks like a nail'

There is a saying in plastic surgery that if the only tool that you have is a hammer, then everything looks like a nail. This means that if you only know one way to do something, then for every problem that you face, you will always try to solve it in the only way you know how. When we are training, we are encouraged to develop our 'reconstructive toolbox', which means that we develop a variety of skills so that we have the knowledge and ability to perform all of the possible operations that could be relevant for a given condition.

When counselling patients about their options for breast reconstruction, I have come across patients who have only been given one surgical option and were not aware of the other options which may have also been suitable. I once saw a patient for a second opinion, who had had a mastectomy following cancer and had been told that she would need to have a breast reduction of her other breast in order to match the size of the breast reconstruction she was about to have. She was not aware that it would have been possible to have a breast reconstruction that could match the size of her breast and this option had not been presented to her. It is true that it was more difficult to match a larger breast and after discussion, she may have chosen to have the reduction anyway (she did not, but went ahead with the more complicated reconstruction to match the size of her breast) but at least she would have gone ahead fully informed of all of the possibilities.

Doctors these days are encouraged to engage with patients about their treatments and their management plan. Nowadays with the internet, patients are more informed than ever. However, the internet can just give the raw information, which can be misleading as it may not be relevant or appropriate for your condition. This is why it is still essential to have a professional opinion on what might be best for you. The beauty of being able to combine the information that is available on the internet, with the considered opinion of a professional, is that you can have an informed discussion about the pros and cons of the various options and how they would relate to you.

Do not be afraid to ask questions and make sure that you reach a management plan that you understand and are comfortable with. You are likely to get a much better outcome if you are engaged with the decision process and you will be better equipped to understand and cope with any complications or unfavourable outcomes if you are fully informed about the risks and benefits of all of the available options.

"You are likely to get a much better outcome if you are engaged with the decision process"

NOTES

NOTES

WHAT IS A PLASTIC SURGEON?

Plastic surgery training is a long haul

Plastic surgery is one of the most competitive surgical specialities. The posts are oversubscribed and there are only a limited number of jobs available in the country.

All plastic surgeons undergo general surgical training first, which will result in the qualification of MRCS and then they need to be accepted onto a higher surgical training scheme which involves six years of specialist training in plastic surgery. This will then lead to the qualification of FRCS(Plast), which indicates that the surgeon is a fully trained specialist.

Not everyone makes it

There is a major bottleneck at the entry to the training schemes and many surgeons will not achieve a place and will have to pursue a different surgical speciality or continue to practice without achieving a specialist qualification. There is no legislation that states that a surgeon needs to have a specialist qualification in order to continue to practice surgery. In the NHS if a surgeon does not have a specialist qualification then they cannot work at a Consultant grade and will need to be supervised by a Consultant. However, in the private sector there is no such ruling and there are many doctors practising in the private sector who have not achieved the level of an NHS Consultant surgeon. Ideally, you should try to find a surgeon who has achieved this level and who is either currently working as a Consultant in the NHS, or has worked as a Consultant in the NHS in the past.

Don't the hospitals check that the surgeons are trained?

The major private hospitals such as BMI, Spire, Ramsay and Nuffield will not allow a surgeon to practice at the hospital if they are not fully trained and this usually means that they have to be or have been a Consultant in the NHS.

However, plastic surgery is one of the few surgical specialities that has commercial providers that offer surgery such as Transform, the Harley Medical Group, MYA and the Hospital Group and these companies have their own hospitals and their own rules. They can employ surgeons who are not NHS Consultants, who may not be eligible to work in one of the major private hospitals but can work in their own hospitals. This means that you may have to travel to one of their hospitals for surgery.

Final examination after at least 15 years of training – FRCS(Plast)

After 5 or 6 years at medical school, a doctor must complete basic surgical training, which takes 3 or 4 years and leads to the qualification of MRCS – Member of the Royal College of Surgeons. Most plastic surgeons then go on to take a higher degree that takes from 1-3 years and will help them to be more competitive when applying for one of the sought after training schemes in plastic surgery. If successful in securing a place on a plastic surgery training scheme, the doctor will then spend six years training in the various fields of plastic surgery under the supervision of a Consultant Plastic Surgeon. Once a surgeon has completed this six years of specialist training, they will be eligible to take an examination which assesses whether they are capable of operating independently. If they are successful in this examination they will be awarded the specialist fellowship in plastic surgery at the Royal College of Surgeons and they will be able to use the letters FRCS(Plast) after their name.

There are only around 400 fully trained plastic surgeons in the UK and so there are many surgeons performing the procedures in which a plastic surgeon is trained who haven't undergone full plastic surgery training.

Plastic surgery is a surgical speciality recognised by the Royal College of Surgeons and there is a structured training scheme and qualification. However, cosmetic surgery is not a surgical speciality in its own right and any surgeon can call themselves a cosmetic surgeon. For that matter there is no restriction on anyone calling themselves a plastic surgeon and there are surgeons who may be considered to be plastic surgeons by their patients who are not actually fully trained in the speciality.

Surely you have to be fully trained to perform surgery?

Unfortunately not. There are a lot of surgeons who have not completed all of their training and have never been a Consultant Plastic Surgeon in the NHS, who are working independently without any supervision.

The minimum requirements to perform surgery are very basic. A doctor has to be fully registered with the GMC in order to practice medicine and prescribe drugs, but this is achieved a year after leaving medical school. There is no requirement for a surgeon to have completed the 10 years or more of specialist training in order to get on the specialist register with the GMC (this can be checked on the GMC website www.gmc-uk.org) and it is up to you, the patient, to make sure that your surgeon is fully trained in the speciality that you think he or she is trained in, i.e. plastic surgery.

There are some high profile cases of celebrities suffering complications following plastic surgery who later discovered that their surgeons were not plastic surgeons and may not have even been a surgeon at all. I have no doubt that these celebrities thought that their surgeons were fully qualified, but it is easy to be blinded by glossy brochures and impressive marketing.

How can I check?

If the surgeon is or has been a Consultant Plastic Surgeon in the NHS or has the letters FRCS(Plast) after their name then you can be assured that they are a fully trained plastic surgeon. Alternatively, you can look at the GMC website at www.gmc-uk.org and click on 'check a doctor's registration'. Here you can see if the doctor is on the specialist register and what surgical speciality they are a specialist in. You will also be able to see if there are any concerns about their fitness to practice.

OK, so my surgeon is fully trained in plastic surgery and has the FRCS(Plast), so I should be fine, right?

Yes, that is right, you should be fine and most plastic surgeons will have a broad training focussing on the restoration of form and function and can turn their hands to most of the more common cosmetic procedures. However, surgeons are increasingly becoming more specialised, and so it is advisable to find a plastic surgeon who has gone on to sub-specialise in breast surgery if you are considering cosmetic breast surgery.

Sub-specialities in Plastic Surgery

Towards the end of plastic surgery training, if the surgeon has done well, they will tend to undergo sub-speciality training in a particular area which will involve working in a unit with a national or international reputation in order to hone their skills in their chosen field of specialisation. Once the surgeon has specialised in plastic surgery they will then need to choose a sub-speciality interest. The subspecialities of plastic surgery are as follows:

- Hand surgery
- Head & neck reconstruction
- Skin cancer surgery
- Cleft and craniofacial surgery
- Burns surgery
- Breast reconstruction

Note, there is no sub-speciality of cosmetic surgery. If your surgeon has an NHS practice, then the majority of their work will be in their sub-speciality field. In fact, it is becoming increasingly difficult for surgeons to maintain a general interest and they will not be allowed to operate in the NHS in a field that they do not have sub-speciality training in. For instance, a hand surgeon will not be allowed to do breast reconstruction.

The NHS is more tightly controlled than the private sector

You may think that if you were to pay privately to see a doctor, then you would be assured of seeing someone with at least as good as, and if not better, qualifications than an NHS doctor, but this is not necessarily the case. In the private sector it is not uncommon for a surgeon to perform a facelift one day and a breast enlargement the next - something that would not be allowed in the NHS.

In the NHS, you would be under the care of a fully trained Consultant, although you may not necessarily be treated by the Consultant, as there will be a team of junior doctors who will also be looking after you. In the private sector, your care is much more likely to be Consultant-led and you tend not to see any junior doctors. However, you need to make sure that your Consultant is up to the same level of training and expertise as an NHS Consultant. You can find out if your surgeon has a sub-speciality interest by looking at their profile or by asking them.

CASE STUDY

If it can happen to them...

The wealthy rapper Kanye West's mother and manager, Donda West, had breast surgery and an abdominoplasty in 2007 and suffered fatal complications following this. It subsequently transpired that her surgeon was not a board certified plastic surgeon. A board certified plastic surgeon in the USA is equivalent to a surgeon with FRCS(Plast) in the UK. The American Society of Plastic Surgery (ASPS) goes to great lengths to educate the public to look for a fully trained surgeon in the same way that the British Association of Aesthetic Plastic Surgeons (BAAPS) campaigns in the UK to raise awareness of surgical training. However, if someone with the means of Kanye West can fall into this trap, anyone can, and he is not alone.

The wife of the pop star Usher, Tameka Foster-Raymond, suffered a cardiac arrest prior to undergoing abdominal liposuction in 2009. She had travelled from America to Brazil to have her surgery and had given birth to her second son, only two months earlier. Both the overseas flight and having recently given birth are risk factors and so she was increasing her risk by choosing to go abroad for surgery. Furthermore, it appears that her surgeon was not a member of the American Society of Plastic Surgeons either, which reinforces the fact that it is important to do your research and it is all too easy to be seduced by glossy advertising or marketing, without properly researching the surgeon's credentials.

There is a regular stream of stories in the media of patients undergoing plastic surgery treatments and suffering complications from inadequate patient selection, inappropriate products or facilities, or insufficient after-care. The focus of many commercial providers of plastic surgery is often on the glossy results and outcomes rather than the training and experience of the surgeon. Always try to look at the facts. Check the training, look at reviews and ask to speak with previous patients to get a feel of how your chosen surgeon and clinic treats patients – especially after they have had surgery.

You should make sure that you meet with your surgeon before surgery and have the time and space to ask him or her as many questions as you like. We always encourage a second consultation before going ahead with surgery and you should be able to feel like you can contact the clinic with any questions or concerns no matter how trivial or insignificant you feel they might be.

This is a major life event and you need to feel comfortable in your own mind that all of your questions have been answered. You need to make sure that you have a good connection with your surgeon and you need to be allowed enough access to him or her to enable you to make a connection. It is not necessary that you like your surgeon, but alarm bells should ring if you feel that you *dislike* your surgeon. You should feel comfortable asking your surgeon questions about his or her training, experience and qualifications. If you find that they are evasive or uncomfortable tackling these questions – this should be a warning sign. Most surgeons who are fully trained in plastic surgery will be only too happy to talk about their experience and will be proud of their qualifications.

"This is a major life event and you need to feel comfortable in your own mind that all of your questions have been answered"

NOTES

NOTES

DOES TRAINING MATTER?

The benchmark of surgical training is when a surgeon becomes an NHS Consultant. This is the pinnacle of a surgeon's career and if a surgeon is or has been an NHS Consultant, then this gives the reassurance that they have completed their training and have been assessed to be capable of operating and managing patients independently. If it is not obvious when reading a surgeon's biography whether they are or have been an NHS Consultant, then they probably have never been one. If you are unsure, it is perfectly reasonable to ask them.

There are many surgeons operating within the private sector who have not completed specialist training and would not be eligible to work as a Consultant in the NHS. One of the problems with the cosmetic industry is the lack of transparency when it comes to training, qualifications and experience and it is all too easy for a doctor to appear qualified with a well written biography, when in fact they are not. It may be perfectly reasonable for that doctor to be providing their services and they may be getting excellent results with lots of happy patients, so does training matter?

We have formal training programs in surgery for a reason. It is a way to ensure that everybody has reached a minimum standard to be able to deliver care in a safe and ethical way. This is not to say that surgeons who have not achieved this level of training cannot still provide a good service, but there is not the safety net that is present with trained doctors.

Fully trained doctors will be accountable to their professional bodies. For plastic surgeons, there is the British Association of Plastic, Reconstructive and Aesthetic Surgeons (BAPRAS) and the British Association of Aesthetic Plastic Surgeons (BAAPS). Only fully trained plastic surgeons are able to become members of these associations and we are bound to a code of conduct and held accountable to our peers.

Why do I need to go away for my surgery?

If your surgeon is fully trained, then you will probably be able to have your surgery close to home, which is always preferable. This is because the major private providers in the UK, such as BMI, Spire, Ramsay and Nuffield Hospitals are located in and around most major towns and cities. However, they will only allow surgeons who have finished their training to work there. So if you are looking for a surgeon, then a good place to start is to talk to your local private hospital.

We also have cosmetic surgery companies in the UK and these employ surgeons who are not fully trained and so they are limited in the hospitals which they can work in. This has led some commercial clinics to open their own hospitals to give an environment in which their surgeons are able to practice. However, there will only be one or two of these facilities in the country, which means that you may need to travel to get to these hospitals for your surgery and this can be inconvenient and can cause other problems (see surgery overseas chapter).

Word of mouth recommendation

It is all very well having the qualifications but does it matter? I say to patients or friends who are considering having any procedure that personal recommendation is always a great way to choose a practitioner. This goes for other walks of life too – plumbers, builders and accountants all rely on recommendation and the good ones will make sure that their customers are happy because they realise the importance of good customer service. My practice relies heavily on word of mouth recommendation and I realise this is a major reason why people come to see me. However, while word of mouth is an excellent way to help to choose which surgeon or clinic to go to, it is also important to be aware of the credentials of the surgeon or clinic in the same way that you should know the credentials of your builder or accountant.

It is not always easy to find someone who can recommend a surgeon because, while cosmetic surgery is much more open and accepted these days, there is still an undertone of guilt and taboo associated with it. For this reason, you may not know anyone who has had surgery and so may be unable to get a recommendation.

The next step would be to go to your General Practitioner as he or she will recommend a local plastic surgeon who will be sure to be fully trained as they are likely to have an NHS Consultant practice. However, many people don't like to see their General Practitioner as they feel that they may not want them to know and they may feel that it is not relevant to them.

For these reasons, the most common way that someone will choose a surgeon is by looking on the Internet and at marketing materials. It is good that there is so much information available these days but it is important to be able to see through glossy advertising and look at the facts relating to the qualifications and credentials of the surgeon and the facility that is offering the treatment. The facts can sometimes be difficult to find and is one of the reasons that I have written this book.

Once you have found an appropriately trained surgeon the next step is to meet them. Do not underestimate the importance of developing a rapport with your surgeon. It is important that you have a good line of communication and that you feel you will be listened to and looked after. Cosmetic surgery is a very subjective field and it is important that you are able to get your point across to make sure that the result is what you are hoping to achieve. It is equally important for the surgeon to feel that they are able to make you understand what is achievable so that you are both on the same page. You should be able to go back to your surgeon for a second consultation before embarking on a procedure and in fact I encourage this with my patients. There should be no pressure or incentive to proceed with surgery as this is a medical procedure and if it is right for you, you should not need to be incentivised to go ahead with it. If your surgeon is a fully trained plastic surgeon, he or she will likely be a member of the British Association of Aesthetic Plastic Surgeons (the BAAPS) who have a code of conduct which does not allow the use of incentives or time-limited offers.

If you do not feel that you are able to develop a rapport with your surgeon or you do not feel that you have been given enough time to go through things prior to surgery, then you should not feel that you need to proceed. You should be allowed the time and the space to make an informed decision – there are many fully trained surgeons in the country and I would encourage you to seek a second, third, or however many opinions you need until you are comfortable.

CASE STUDY

Do not assume you are seeing a plastic surgeon

I was approached by a tax accountant who offered to help me with my financial affairs. He offered a free initial consultation and then said he would need to come back for a second visit to go over things in more detail. He wanted me to sign some forms on the second visit to give him control over my financial matters and I did not feel comfortable with this. He was quite assertive and I did not have a good feeling about him. I am ashamed to say that I signed the forms just to get him to leave the house, but I was not comfortable with the whole interaction.

On reflection, I decided that I did not want to have this man working on my affairs and so I contacted his office to cancel the arrangement. He then sent me a bill for £700 for the second consultation. I pointed out that this was on his suggestion and I had not wanted a second consultation (to be honest, I did not like him after the first consultation). I felt that he had not acted professionally and had not been transparent about charging for the second consultation. I contacted the professional associations for accountants, only to find that he was not a member of either of the established associations. He was not a qualified chartered accountant and as such, was not bound to work within any established guidelines or principles. He needed to work within the law, but there were no professional or ethical guidelines that he was bound to.

I pointed out to the professional accountancy associations that they need to educate the public more about what to look out for in your accountant as I had been duped into thinking that this man was a qualified accountant. I then realised that we have the same problem with plastic surgery.

There are two professional associations for plastic surgeons – The British Association of Plastic, Reconstructive and Aesthetic Surgeons (BAPRAS) and The British Association of Aesthetic Plastic Surgeons (BAAPS). They have strict entry criteria and professional guidelines that we all have to work within. As a member, we need to submit an annual audit of the numbers of operations performed and any complications or re-operations.

If your surgeon is not a member of one of the plastic surgery associations, then they will not be bound by the strict guidelines that plastic surgeons are held to. However, all doctors are accountable to the General Medical Council (the GMC) and the GMC have now put out guidelines for cosmetic surgery that all doctors should work within. I was asked to comment on these guidelines by the BBC and I was delighted that they had been produced, but they were guidelines that any BAAPS member had been working within for some time. They included things like allowing patients a 2 week 'cooling off' period between consultation and surgery and not allowing time limited offers or 'buy one get one free' deals. This is an effort to bring the other doctors performing cosmetic surgery into line with the standards demanded of plastic surgeons. Be aware that this protection only covers medically qualified doctors, so if you are treated by a non-medically trained practitioner, then you will not have the same level of protection.

"If your surgeon is not a member of one of the plastic surgery associations – BAPRAS or BAAPS, then they will not be bound by the strict guidelines that plastic surgeons are held to"

NOTES

NOTES

IS TRAINING THE SAME ACROSS SPECIALITIES?

All surgical training is based within the NHS and it varies quite widely across specialities. There are no formal surgical training schemes within the private sector, although there are fellowships and observer posts.

The NHS has a structure for medical training

All doctors will have undergone training within the health service. There is a well-defined structure and pathway for doctors to go through as they progress with their medical training. All doctors will have undertaken a medical degree which will take between five or six years in University after leaving school and lead to the award of MBBS or MB ChB after their name. When a doctor leaves medical school, he or she will be able to use the title Dr. and after a year of working in a hospital, will be fully registered with the General Medical Council (GMC) and will be able to prescribe drugs.

After basic training in the hospital for two years, the doctor will be encouraged to choose an area of medicine to work in. This will involve either training to become a GP, training to become a physician or training to become a surgeon. Surgical training is different from the other two in that there are two major sets of exams rather than one because there is a period of speciality training culminating in an exit examination.

GP training takes about four years and it takes about six years to become a physician. There are exams to take at the beginning of the training to enter the Royal Colleges. For GP it is the MRCGP (Member of the Royal College of General Practitioners) and for physicians, it is the MRCP (Member of the Royal College of Physicians) and you will see these letters after the doctor's name.

Surgical training requires two exams

Surgical training is different in that there are two exams to take. One at the beginning of the training and one at the end. The first exam is the MRCS which stands for Member of the Royal College of Surgeons (it used to be called the FRCS, which is a Fellow of the College, so older surgeons will have FRCS). The second exam is the specialist fellowship and the speciality will be signified in brackets after the letters FRCS, eg FRCS(Plast) – this exam is taken at the end of the training.

A doctor needs to have done at least two years of surgical training in various specialities to be eligible to take the first exam to become a member of the college. The exam tests basic surgical knowledge across all of the surgical disciplines and can take several years to pass it. Once the MRCS exam has been passed then the doctor can use the title Mr. He or she will also be able to apply for a higher surgical training scheme which is a five or six-year post during which the doctor will be supervised in their chosen surgical speciality and will lead to them becoming a specialist.

Plastic surgery is one of the more oversubscribed training schemes and in order to gain a place, a doctor, will often have to have a higher degree such as a master's degree (MSc, MD) or a doctorate (PhD) and this will take between 1-3 years of full-time study. At the end of the training scheme there will be the exit examination to take, which is designed to test whether the surgeon is capable of operating independently. Only then will the surgeon be considered to be a specialist and will be eligible to hold a specialist fellowship with the Royal College of Surgeons. You will be able to tell because the doctor will have the letters of the speciality in brackets after the FRCS after their name, such as FRCS(Plast) for plastic surgery, FRCS(Gen) for general surgery, FRCS(Orth) for orthopaedic surgery and so on.

This means that it can take anything from 10-15 years of postgraduate training to become a fully trained surgeon in one of the surgical disciplines.

The focus of the training obviously depends on the area of surgery that is being pursued. The focus of plastic surgery training is on reconstruction and aesthetics. There are different fields within plastic surgery – head and neck cancer, breast, skin, burns, hands and paediatric plastic surgery. The common theme to the training is meticulous attention to tissue handling and minimising trauma while operating. Plastic surgeons are experts in wound care and healing and if another surgeon has a problem with a wound in the hospital, they call a plastic surgeon for advice and help in managing it.

Training by speciality

There are many different specialists who perform cosmetic surgery and the main groups are listed below:

General Practitioner (GP)

General Practitioners have a shortened training scheme compared to surgeons. They have a wide breadth of experience and there is a separate GP register with the GMC for you to check whether your GP has finished their training (enter the name or GMC number of your doctor in the 'check your doctor's credentials section of the GMC website and it will say if they are on the GP register). There is no formal surgical training for General Practitioners. Some GPs go on to do extra training and can perform non-surgical treatments and they are known as cosmetic doctors.

Dermatologist

Dermatologists have medical training but are not part of any of the surgical colleges as they have no formal surgical training. Dermatologists are experts in the management of skin conditions and frequently perform minor surgical procedures under local anaesthetic such as removal of moles and cysts. Some dermatologists will also perform non-surgical cosmetic treatments.

ENT surgeon / Maxillofacial surgeon / General surgeon

These are surgical specialities and are part of the Royal College of Surgeons. You can check whether a surgeon is fully trained in one of these specialities on the GMC website (www.gmc-org.uk) as they will be on the specialist register in their given speciality. These specialists will usually have NHS Consultant posts and may also perform cosmetic surgery, but it will be important to see what the majority of their work and training is to check whether they will be appropriate to do your procedure. For instance, it is perfectly reasonable for an ENT (ears, nose and throat) surgeon to perform a rhinoplasty (nose job), but you may want to reconsider if he or she was to offer to put in breast implants. You can tell which speciality your surgeon is trained in by the letters in brackets after FRCS after their name.

FRCS (ORL) – ENT surgeon

FRCS (OMFS) – Maxillofacial surgeon

FRCS (Gen) – General surgeon

Plastic surgeon

Cosmetic or aesthetic surgery is a major component of plastic surgery and plastic surgery is the only surgical speciality with this as a significant part of the training. Most plastic surgeons will have a sub-speciality interest and so you should ask what this is as it could be burn surgery or hand surgery. Only a subset of plastic surgeons will have sub-speciality training in breast surgery. There is currently no sub-speciality of cosmetic surgery.

All of the specialists listed above may be performing cosmetic procedures with good outcomes - just because someone is not a fully trained plastic surgeon, it does not mean you will have a poor outcome. However, it is important that you go into any surgical procedure with your eyes open and fully informed about the training and experience of your surgeon.

CASE STUDY

You may need to dig to find the truth

One of the problems with cosmetic surgery is that people tend to treat it with less diligence than they would for other surgical procedures. The reasons for patients to choose a surgeon or a clinic are often based on quite superficial criteria like the advertising or how nice the nurse (or salesperson) was when they went to the clinic (who may be on commission and who they may never see again).

For some reason, they do not approach it in the same way that they would if they were having another procedure, such as a hip replacement or a brain tumour removed. If you were having a hip replacement, there is no way that you would consider anyone other than an orthopaedic surgeon doing your procedure and it you had a brain tumour, you would want a neurosurgeon (brain surgeon). You would not want the orthopaedic surgeon to do your brain surgery and you wouldn't let the brain surgeon touch your hip. So why do people let all types of surgeons do plastic surgery on them?

This industry often does a good job of hiding the qualifications of the surgeons and it is up to you to do some digging to find out exactly what training and experience your surgeon has. I think that many people take it for granted that all of the surgeons will be plastic surgeons and are often shocked to hear how few plastic surgeons there are in the country.

I was asked for a second opinion by a patient who had had correction of gynaecomastia at a national clinic and he was unhappy with the result. I asked who his surgeon was and he mentioned a name that I had not heard of. I asked if he was a plastic surgeon and the patient confirmed that he thought it was a plastic surgeon. Because the plastic surgery community is quite small, I usually know or know of most of the plastic surgeons in the country. On closer investigation it turned out that the surgeon's training was in Accident & Emergency medicine. There is no formal surgical training involved in Accident & Emergency medicine, however, this patient was under the impression that his surgeon was a plastic surgeon. In fact, reading the surgeon's biography on the website, it gave the impression that he was a plastic surgeon, so I understand why the patient thought what he did.

The information is freely available, but you have to dig to find it and you have to know where to dig. In this case, the surgeon had provided his GMC number in his biography (which we are all encouraged to do) and a search on the GMC website (www.gmc-org.uk) revealed what he had been trained in. Alternatively, just look for the letters FRCS(Plast) after their name.

"You would not want the orthopaedic surgeon to do brain surgery and you wouldn't let the brain surgeon touch your hip. So why do people let all types of surgeons do plastic surgery on them?"

NOTES

NOTES

IS TRAINING THE SAME ACROSS COUNTRIES?

There are many excellent surgeons all over the world and no country can claim to have the best surgical training. However, the UK has an enviable reputation for producing fully trained Consultant Surgeons who possess the decision making capabilities and surgical skills to be able to operate independently without senior supervision.

Every country has its own way of training surgeons

Other countries have different surgical hierarchies and even though a surgeon may be fully trained, they will often still operate under the supervision of a 'chief' or 'professor'. Overseas doctors who are fully trained in their own country, will often come to the UK for further training in their specialist field. It is not that the training is of any less quality than UK training, but training schemes overseas are variable and cover different areas and to varying degrees of depth. For instance, plastic surgery training in the USA does not involve any of the immediate management of burn injuries, whereas this is an integral part of the training in the UK. Similarly, plastic surgery training in Italy does not cover the management of hand injuries, whereas this is comprehensively covered in the training in the UK. On the flip side, plastic surgery training in Australia and New Zealand has aspects to it that cover maxillofacial surgery in greater depth than the training in the UK. It is the fact that the training around the world is variable that makes it difficult to be sure to what level a surgeon has reached if they are to come to the UK to practice.

In the UK, a Consultant post in the NHS is the pinnacle of a surgeon's training

Once surgeons have finished plastic surgery training in the UK (when they have achieved the FRCS(Plast) qualification), they are eligible to apply for a Consultant post in the NHS. This is seen as the pinnacle of a doctor's training in this country, and until a doctor has achieved the Consultant grade, they will not be able to operate in the NHS unless they are under the supervision of a Consultant. In medical terms, they are junior doctors until they have achieved a Consultant post and become senior doctors. However, there are many surgeons operating in the private sector who have never been an NHS Consultant and would not be eligible to operate independently in the NHS without further training, yet they are free to operate independently in the private system. In the NHS they would be considered a junior doctor.

The term 'junior doctor' does not refer to the doctor's age; it refers to whether a doctor has finished their training or not. A doctor will typically achieve a senior role (ie a Consultant post) around the age of 35-40 and many will never achieve it.

In the private system, a doctor is free to operate and perform surgery unsupervised, even though they would not be allowed to do so in the NHS – it may sound unbelievable, but it is true and it is happening. The NHS has a rigorous and comprehensive process for vetting surgeons before becoming a Consultant, and so if a surgeon from overseas has come to the UK and achieved a Consultant post in the NHS, then you can be reassured that they have attained a certain level of training. However, for those that do not have any such measure of their experience, it can be difficult to judge how comprehensive the training has been.

Be aware of where your surgeon has been trained

In the UK, there are several companies that provide cosmetic surgery. These companies are not so prevalent overseas and in other parts of Europe where the majority of the work is done by the 'professor' or 'chief' of the department. This makes it difficult for surgeons overseas who have not achieved the level of training of the professor or chief to build up an independent practice of their own.

The cosmetic surgery companies allow surgeons from other countries to come to the UK to operate without having an established practice or reputation of their own. If the surgeon has not completed surgical training to the level of a Consultant, they will not be allowed to operate in any of the major private hospitals in the UK, such as Spire,

BMI, Nuffield and Ramsay, and so the companies have to have their own hospitals in which their surgeons can operate.

This has a couple of limitations. Firstly, these hospitals will often only provide plastic surgery services whereas the major private hospitals in the UK all have a much broader range of specialities represented. The benefit of having doctors from other specialities working in the same hospital is that it becomes very easy to get an opinion if you have a problem outside the scope of plastic surgery, such as palpitations or breathing problems. If you have surgery in a hospital where the relevant specialist is not available, then you may find yourself in an ambulance going to the local A&E department.

The other problem with the company owning hospitals is that they are limited in number and you may find yourself having to travel long distances for your surgery. This can be inconvenient and it is not ideal to have a long journey immediately after surgery and can also make it difficult for friends and family to visit you. Furthermore, if you were to require any revision surgery you would have to travel again. I will talk further about the problems of having surgery far away from home in the next chapter.

CASE STUDY

The Law Is Not On Your Side

There was a recent news article about a practitioner who was performing non-surgical injections on patients at house parties and in unlicensed premises. It turns out that he used to be a psychiatric nurse but got struck off the nursing register following allegations of misconduct with one of his patients.

The story was presented as an exposé of this dodgy practitioner who was seen as a rogue nurse. However, I have spoken to patients who had been treated by him and they knew that he used to be a nurse as he freely offered this information and so what he was doing was not illegal. You may say "there may not be a law against it, but what about the guidelines?" The problem is that he was not bound by any guidelines because he did not belong to any professional association. When you read the story, you would be shocked that this man was treating patients, but when you read between the lines, you realise that he was not actually doing much wrong. From a medical point of view, the only thing that he was doing wrong was prescribing Botox when he did not have a license to prescribe, and if this was the case, the pharmacist who was filling his prescriptions should also be held to account. There are many people out there performing non-surgical treatments who are not qualified to prescribe the treatments and who get doctors to make out prescriptions on their behalf. This is known as 'remote prescribing' and, whilst it is frowned upon, it does go on and it allows people with no medical qualifications to perform non-surgical injections.

It is important to point out that whilst only qualified medical practitioners – doctors, dentists and specially qualified nurses (nurse prescribers) – can prescribe drugs such as Botox, there is no regulation on who can inject it. Worse still, products such as dermal fillers are not even classified as medicines so you do not need a prescription, which means that anyone can get their hands on them and inject them – your hairdresser, your beautician, even your neighbour.

The shocking thing about this story is that anyone can perform these treatments with no qualifications whatsoever and there is no legislation or guidelines against this. This means that it is more important than ever for you to do your own research and make sure that you know what qualifications and training your practitioner has had. You need to do your research and don't be afraid to ask questions.

"The real story is that anyone can perform these treatments with no qualifications whatsoever and there is no legislation or guidelines against this"

NOTES

NOTES

SURGERY OVERSEAS (OR FAR FROM HOME)

I can see the attraction in having surgery overseas. Not only is the cost of the surgery often cheaper than the cost in the UK, but there is also the added benefit of having a trip abroad which could be thought of as a holiday.

However, beware, as the training of surgeons overseas is variable (see previous chapter) and it can be difficult to tell when one has reached the equivalent level of a Consultant Plastic Surgeon in the UK and achieved the required level of training to be operating without supervision. The terminology can be different in that in some European countries the terms 'professor' and 'associate professor' are used more widely than they are in the UK. Here in the UK we only have a handful of professors in plastic surgery and it signifies a position in which the doctor will have a significant academic aspect to their day to day work and be involved in research or training.

You get what you pay for?

You have to ask yourself 'why is surgery so much cheaper overseas?' The amount that surgeons need to pay for their medical indemnity insurance overseas is often significantly less than what a surgeon in the UK would have to pay. This means that if you do suffer harm or find the need to seek legal action against the doctor, they may not be able to cover the costs of a claim to the same level. This also applies to overseas doctors working in the UK. They may have indemnity insurance in their own country, which may not cover to the same level that is required in most private hospitals in the UK. If you are treated in one of the major private hospitals, such as Spire, BMI, Nuffield and Ramsay, then you can rest assured that your surgeon will be obliged to have sufficient medical insurance. However, some of the cosmetic chains employ overseas surgeons who would not be eligible to work in one of the major hospitals because of their qualifications and so they have set up their own hospitals, which may not have the same level of insurance requirements.

Will I see my doctor again?

You should check the level of support and aftercare given. The support and aftercare given to patients following surgery is the most important aspect of my practice, yet is something that patients often do not consider.

Fortunately, complications and unfavourable results are rare in cosmetic surgery; however, it is important for you to know that there will be help available to you should you need it. Problems can range from significant complications, which may require a return to the operating theatre, to minor twinges, aches or bulges, which may require observation and reassurance, preferably from the surgeon. It is important that there is someone you can contact and somewhere you can go 24 hours a day, 365 days a year if you need help. Ideally you should have access to your surgeon and, failing that, any doctor who sees you post operatively should have your notes, including a copy of your operating notes with the post-operative instructions and have access to your surgeon for advice and guidance.

It is always best to see the surgeon who operated on you when you have any questions or concerns about your procedure. Scars, bruising and swelling always take time to settle and the degree of settling is often variable. Very frequently, reassurance is all that is required and it is always nice if you see the same person at each follow-up appointment so they can more accurately chart your progress. On the rare occasion that you need emergency medical assistance, which might be in the form of an urgent appointment with the doctor, possibly a scan or even further surgery, how should you go about accessing this, and who will pay for it? These are questions that you should be asking the surgeon or the hospital where you are having the surgery so that you know exactly what to do, should the need arise.

If you have some asymmetries or concerns about your result which may require a revision or tidy up procedure, where will this be performed? Will you need to go back overseas to have the surgery, and if so will you have to pay again? This not only relates to the hospital and the surgical fees, but also your flights, travel and hotel expenses. This may also apply if you are having surgery in this country if the hospital is not close to home.

Risk of the Flight

There is another reason to avoid travelling long distances for your surgery. Aside from the inconvenience of getting to and from the hospital, both for you and your family and friends, there is a medical reason to avoid long journeys around the time of surgery.

"Economy class syndrome"

Any period of immobility can lead to clots forming in your legs that can fly off into your lungs, which is a potentially fatal complication of any surgery. The clots that can form in your legs are known as deep vein thromboses (DVT) and if they fly off in to your lungs, then they are known as pulmonary emboli (PE). There are other risk factors for these clots to form such as long periods of travel, particularly in cramped conditions which might make it difficult to exercise your legs to keep the blood flowing - so-called "economy class syndrome". Hence, if you must fly overseas to have your surgery, then you are multiplying your risk of this potentially serious complication.

CASE STUDY

Sun, Sea and Surgery

Unfortunately, when patients have problems after having had surgery abroad, they turn to their local hospitals for help when they get home. The NHS has had to pick up the bill to treat countless cases of botched surgery from abroad, but they will only treat you for an emergency. They will not help if you are simply unhappy with your result or have a non-urgent problem like swelling or asymmetry.

I saw a patient who had had a tummy tuck in Prague several months before and was suffering from recurrent seroma. This is a rare (but not unheard of) complication of tummy tucks where fluid collects in your tummy and needs to be drained off with a needle. Normally this is a relatively straightforward procedure that can be performed in the clinic and it gradually resolves naturally. Unfortunately for this lady, it kept coming back when it was drained and she needed a surgical procedure to remove the swelling, which she had to go back to Prague for. I was seeing her because the swelling had come back despite the revision surgery and she was at the end of her tether. The costs of returning to Prague to see her surgeon and an overnight stay to have the surgery, were not factored in when she originally budgeted for the procedure, not to mention the stress and anxiety of not having regular contact with her surgeon.

These problems are rare, but it is not uncommon to have a minor bulge or bump that you may be concerned about and you may just need reassurance from your surgeon, so I would always advise patients to have surgery close to home if they can. Even when I get enquiries from around the country, I would always say that it is probably better to have surgery closer to home for the peace of mind that is afforded by having your surgeon close at hand. Of course, we have email, phone and Skype to keep in touch, but there is no substitute for a face to face meeting.

"The NHS has had to pick up the bill to treat countless cases of botched surgery from abroad"

Never Accept a Lift from Strangers

Jonathan Staiano

WHO IS THE BEST BREAST SURGEON?

Like most things in life, there is no straight answer to who is the best; it depends on what you need. There are two types of consultants who specialise in breast surgery (see chapter 1) and these can be difficult to tell apart, unless you know what you are looking for. There is the breast surgeon who has gone through general surgery training and will have FRCS(Gen) after their name, and there is the plastic surgeon who has gone through plastic surgery training and will have FRCS(Plast) after their name.

The best type of surgeon to treat you will depend on the problem that you have.

If you have a breast lump

If you have:
- A breast lump or cancer worries
- Breast pain
- Nipple disease or discharge

Then a General Surgeon will be the best port of call for you. This is the surgeon who you will be referred to in the NHS if you have a breast problem and they are experts in the treatment of breast cancer, performing lumpectomies, mastectomies and coordinating the treatment and follow up after removal of your cancer.

If you need breast reconstruction

If you need:

- Breast reconstruction following a mastectomy or wide local excision of a breast lump

Then traditionally, you would have seen a plastic surgeon for this, but some general breast surgeons have gone on to spend time (usually one or two years) with plastic surgeons to train in the techniques required for breast reconstruction, and these are known as 'oncoplastic breast surgeons'. They may not be able to perform all of the different methods of breast reconstruction, but they can offer the majority, and if you need a reconstruction that they cannot perform, they will usually have a plastic surgeon that they can refer you to for this. Usually, the breast surgeon will only perform the reconstruction of your breast and if you need any balancing surgery on the other breast, then you may be referred to a plastic surgeon for this. This can take the form of a breast reduction, a breast lift or a breast enlargement.

If you need cosmetic surgery

If you need:

- A breast enlargement
- A breast reduction
- A breast lift

Then any plastic surgeon will probably be able to perform this, and most plastic surgeons will offer these treatments, regardless of their speciality interest because there is a common theme of aesthetics throughout plastic surgery training. In more difficult cases, such as if you have an asymmetry or are very slim, or if you need a large breast reduction, then it may be beneficial to choose a plastic surgeon with a special interest in the breast, but in most cases any plastic surgeon will be able to offer surgery.

There are other types of surgeon that offers this sort of surgery, such as general breast surgeons and if they have undergone a period of training with a plastic surgeon (oncoplastic surgeons), then they may be able to offer this surgery too.

If you have a breast asymmetry

If you have:

- A complex breast deformity or asymmetry

Then a plastic surgeon with a special interest in the breast would be the best option for you. These cases may require changes in the shape and the structure of the breast and often have common themes with breast reconstruction after mastectomy. They may involve complex techniques to recreate the shape of the inframammary fold (the fold where the bra sits) and making sure that the size and the proportion of the breast is matched and balanced.

You may require further work on your nipple and/or areola and your surgery may need to be done in stages which requires careful planning and support.

CASE STUDY

Make sure that you are offered all of the options

I have seen countless patients who have previously seen other surgeons and been to other clinics. I always talk about polyurethane foam coated breast implants as an option, as they have some significant benefits and I give my patients the opportunity to decide whether they might be right for them. Most patients have never heard of these implants before. This is probably because the other surgeons or clinics do not use them and so do not talk about them. However, as doctors, we are encouraged to give patients all of the available options for treatment to allow you to make a balanced and informed decision. If you are not told about these implants, then you are not being given the choice.

This is why it is important to see a specialist. A surgeon who treats a condition only occasionally and does not specialise in it, may have limited experience and a limited repertoire. You should be offered a balanced overview of all of the available options to treat a given condition and this requires the expertise of a specialist, ideally one who is independent and can offer you everything so that you can decide what is right for you. Ask questions and if you feel resistance or get evasive answers, then seek a second opinion.

"You should be offered a balanced overview of all of the available options to treat a given condition and this requires the expertise of a specialist"

NOTES

NOTES

INDIVIDUAL SURGEON vs COMPANY

Commercial Cosmetic Clinics

In the UK, we have many commercial companies that provide cosmetic surgery. This is not the case in America or other parts of Europe where the majority of plastic surgery is performed by fully trained, independent plastic surgeons. The commercial companies are strong on sales and marketing and they have a national reach with a big advertising budget. They tend not to put the surgeon front and centre and use a variety of surgeons from different specialities with different levels of training. Many of the surgeons would not be eligible to hold an NHS Consultant post and so would not qualify to work in one of the major private hospitals (BMI, Spire, Ramsay, BUPA and Nuffield) that are located in most cities throughout the country. This means that the companies need to have their own hospitals to allow their surgeons to operate. This limits the geographical location of where you can have your surgery as they only have one or two hospitals in the country.

The other limitation with this is that their hospitals are typically only performing the more commercial specialities such as cosmetic surgery, weight loss surgery and eye surgery. This means that if you have any postoperative complications with your heart rate or breathing, for instance, and need to see a specialist, you may need to be transferred to the local A&E department. Your local private hospital, however, will have all of the specialities represented with consultants on hand for help or an opinion should you develop any problems that are outside the expertise of the surgeon who is looking after you. Some of the more major private hospitals even have intensive care units on site, and whilst it is extremely unlikely you will need this, it can be reassuring to know that it is there.

Most of the commercial companies employ patient advisors who will see patients initially and be a point of contact. This is a good idea in principle; however, it can be dangerous to rely too heavily on the advice and recommendations of a practitioner who may not be trained to do the procedure and will not be the one to perform your surgery. There can also be concerns if the advisor is paid by commission that they may not have your best interests at heart.

Having surgery is a significant undertaking and you need to make sure that you have the time and space to make an informed decision and to weigh up the pros and cons of any procedure. Make sure that you are comfortable with your surgeon and that you have the time to get the answers to your questions, preferably from the surgeon themselves.

Independent Plastic Surgeons

Most fully trained plastic surgeons in the UK work as independent practitioners, although they will work in a local private hospital, such as BMI, Spire, Ramsay, BUPA and Nuffield. This means that you should be able to have your surgery close to your home and this will have benefits, both in terms of convenience for you and your family visiting the hospital, but also from a medical point of view to avoid a long journey around the time of your surgery (see Surgery Overseas Chapter). It also has implications if you need any further surgery, as you may need to go back to the hospital for this.

Independent surgeons are not employed by the hospital and this means that individual surgeons manage their own private practice independently. Surgeons are not trained in marketing and do not have the budget to employ sales people and pay for advertising. This means that they are unable to compete when it comes to internet marketing and adverts on Facebook or Google and so they can be difficult to find if you are doing an internet search. The majority of our work comes through word of mouth recommendation or via enquires through the hospital help lines and the focus of our service is very much directed towards giving the best possible outcome to each individual patient rather than on the commercial interests of the business.

You may find that there is more transparency regarding your surgeon's training and qualifications if you go to an independent plastic surgeon and any surgeon should be happy and proud to go through his or her qualifications (start to worry if they are not). All doctors are encouraged to publicise their GMC (General Medical Council) number and you can go to the GMC website (http://www.gmc-uk.org/) to check whether your doctor is registered, and more importantly, whether they are on the GMC Specialist Register for Plastic Surgery (my GMC number is 4117214 by the way).

What About the Aftercare?

The aftercare is the most important part of the service for any patient in my view, but it is frequently overlooked in favour of other factors, such as the cost of the surgery, the type of implants used or the finance packages available. It is important to ask questions about what exactly is included in the aftercare because it can be confusing. If you are having breast implants, then the implants will have a guarantee, but exactly what this covers can be variable.

Guarantees of Implants

Most implants have a lifetime guarantee (some are 10 years) but it is limited as to what this covers. For detailed information about the manufacturer's warranties, ask your surgeon, or contact their website as there is a lot of information online. It usually only covers rupture of the implant, although Nagor and Mentor also cover capsular contracture. It does not cover you if you are unhappy with the size of your implants or if you have wrinkling or rippling or other cosmetic concerns with your implants. It may allow you to change the size of your implants and it may allow you a free replacement of the opposite breast implant. Here are details of what the major manufacturer warranties cover*:

Nagor

Nagor are a major British manufacturer of implants. They offer a lifetime warranty which covers capsular contracture as well as shell failure (rupture). They will also offer a replacement of both implants even if only one has failed and will allow a change in size up to one size above or below your current size.

Allergan

Allergan are based in the United States and they have two ranges of implants. CUI is their budget range and Natrelle is their premium range.

CUI Implants are covered for 10 years in the event of rupture. They are not covered for capsular contracture and the warranty allows a replacement of your implant.

Natrelle Implants have a lifetime warranty. The warranty does not cover capsular contracture, but they do offer financial

details correct at time of writing, June 2016. For full terms and conditions, contact the implant manufacturer

assistance for up to 10 years following your procedure. They will pay £700 towards your hospital costs if the implant is shown to have a manufacturing fault once it is returned to Allergan following removal. They will offer a replacement of both of your implants and you can choose to change the size of the replacement implants if you wish.

Mentor

Mentor are also an American company and they offer a lifetime product replacement. Similar to Allergan, they will pay 1000 euros if the implant is shown to have ruptured within 10 years of implantation, but they will also cover replacement for capsular contracture.

Polytech

Polytech also make polyurethane implants and are made in Germany. They offer an insurance based warranty which offers £1500 per implant towards your hospital costs if you require revision surgery within 2 years of implantation. There is a comprehensive list of the conditions that are covered available from Polytech.

Guarantees covering Hospital Costs

Probably the biggest cost associated with revision surgery is the hospital costs. This includes the cost of the hospital stay, the theatre costs, the surgeon's fees and the anaesthetist's fees. This is an area where there can be some variation and it is an important area to focus on. Most surgery is done under what is known as a fixed price package and it is standard to include 28 or 30 days cover for complications. This means that if you have a complication such as bleeding or an infection during your hospital stay or in the immediate postoperative period, this will be dealt with for no extra charge.

The length and extent of the cover following this can vary. There are usually specific conditions that are covered which revolve around whether the results of the surgery meet expectations. Unfortunately, satisfaction with the procedure is not guaranteed and the decision as to whether the results of the surgery meet expectations usually rests with the surgeon.

You need to see whether investigations such as scans are covered and whether you will be expected to pay for prescriptions. You are usually given medication to take home following surgery, but if you need any further medication, such as painkillers or antibiotics in the weeks and months following your surgery, you may be expected to pay for this.

If you have had surgery with an independent surgeon, you may be concerned that you will not be covered for aftercare if he or she moves away or retires. Most independent surgeons operate at major private hospitals such as BMI, Spire, Ramsay or Nuffield and there will be a responsibility of the hospital to ensure that you are looked after adequately. This means that they may ask another plastic surgeon to take over your care if your surgeon is no longer available. However, this is a valid concern and is worth considering before your surgery.

Guarantees covering Outpatient Consultations

In plastic surgery, unlike other medical specialities, it is common to offer patients free consultations. Most surgeons are keen to see their postoperative results and encourage patients to come back to the clinic for review, but you should make sure that it is your surgeon that you will be seeing during your outpatient visits as he or she will be best placed to assess and advise you on your surgery. There may be a time scale on this, so if you have a problem or concern several years after your surgery, will your surgeon charge you to come back to the clinic for review?

Many independent plastic surgeons do not charge for review appointments whenever they are, as long as they are related to the original surgery. However, there can be a concern if your surgeon moves away or retires, as you will likely need to find another surgeon to look after you, unless your surgeon makes arrangements. It is not uncommon for surgeons to hand over their practices to other surgeons when they retire and so it may be that you will have someone to turn to, but this is not guaranteed.

CASE STUDY

It's all about the aftercare; you never know until you need it

I saw a patient recently who had had breast surgery with one of the commercial cosmetic clinics. She was unhappy with the result and had not been able to see the surgeon properly after the surgery to discuss her concerns. She felt that she had been fobbed off and the clinic was not interested in helping her.

The feedback that I got from this lady was that the company was only really interested in her until she had paid for her procedure and once she had had surgery, she found it hard to get an appointment and to make her concerns heard. She clearly had an unfavourable result and was delighted when I revised it for her but really this is something that should have been dealt with by her original company.

This is not an isolated case and I regularly hear of cases where patients have not felt well looked after following their surgery. This is sad to hear, but unfortunately I can believe it. Many years ago, I used to work for one of the cosmetic clinics when I was starting out and trying to build my practice. The company just wanted me to see new patients and did not want me to follow up. I found it very hard to see my patients postoperatively and even then, I could only see them once. Obviously, the company was focusing on the most cost-effective use of my time and delegating the aftercare to the nurses. However, my view is that aftercare is an integral part of the package and I want to see my patients postoperatively, particularly if they have any questions or concerns.

There are many good surgeons out there delivering excellent service and results, but there are also some who are only interested in operating. I have seen surgeons who may be technically proficient at performing the surgery, but do not have the ethos or commitment to listening to and looking after their patient once the surgery is done. This can lead to patients feeling isolated and let down. In my experience, this is a major cause of dissatisfaction amongst patients.

It is not necessarily the surgical result, but it is the way you are treated after the surgery. Often minor irregularities or asymmetries will settle over time and if not, can be corrected with a simple procedure, but if you feel that you are not being listened to and nurtured through this, then you will be unhappy.

I have heard it said:

"he's a good surgeon, but he is not very good with his patients"

In my view, this is not a good surgeon.

This is all part of treating the patient.

So how do you know if your surgeon will look after you postoperatively? Well, it is possible to get some clues.

It is always good to meet with your surgeon on more than one occasion preoperatively. Not only so that you can go through the surgical plan and make sure your goals match his or hers, but also so that you can get a feeling for them. You need to try to develop a rapport. It is a professional relationship, but you should feel comfortable being able to ask questions and change your mind. There should be open access to your surgeon to go through things before surgery and you should not feel any pressure to proceed. If you have trouble contacting or accessing your surgeon before surgery, then you should be worried that they may be difficult to access postoperatively.

Most plastic surgeons work as sole traders and have their own private practice that they are responsible for. This means that they need to make sure that they look after their patients because it is their business. However, there are many surgeons in this industry who do not run their own practice. These are often those who are not fully UK trained plastic surgeons and they work under the umbrella of a company or cosmetic clinic. They do not have the same level of commitment to your long-term care because they will be paid by the company and you will not pay them directly. You may find that if you have any concerns after surgery, you will be dealing with the company, rather than the surgeon directly and this can lead to dissatisfaction and disappointment.

"I have heard it said:
'he's a good surgeon, but he is not
very good with his patients'
In my view, this is not a good surgeon!"

NOTES

NOTES

WHO AM I TO TALK TO ABOUT THIS?

I am a plastic surgeon with a special interest in cosmetic breast surgery. I spent 18 years working in the NHS and have undergone full specialist training in the UK. My training was mainly in London, the North West and Wales and I was awarded the FRCS(Plast), which is the highest qualification possible for a plastic surgeon, in 2005. I went on to perform specialist fellowships in the field of cancer reconstruction at the Royal Marsden Hospital in London and in Wellington New Zealand. I have spent five years as a Consultant Plastic Surgeon in the NHS, initially in Addenbrooke's Hospital in Cambridge and then at City Hospital in Birmingham where my work was dedicated to breast reconstruction following mastectomy. I left the NHS in 2012 and I set up my own clinic, The Staiano Clinic, in 2013 with the aim of providing the best quality experience to patients, delivered by the most highly trained professionals. The focus of my practice is in delivering the highest levels of service and skill in beautiful surroundings. The Staiano Clinic is a world-class establishment and is at the forefront of a new phase in plastic surgery, where customer care and patient engagement are at the heart of the service. All of the practitioners who work at the clinic are leaders in their field and we all share the same commitments:

The Staiano Commitments

- We will do everything we can to ensure you get the best result possible.

- We will give you the time and space you need to make the right decision for you

- We will go the extra mile to help you and make your experience exceptional.

- We will listen to your feedback and act on this to strive to continually improve our service.

- We will always give you our best advice, which might mean recommending no treatment.

- We will only employ fully trained and ethical surgeons and practitioners who share our brand values.

- We will pay attention to detail in everything that we do.

BONUS

Visit www.neveracceptaliftfromstrangers.com to receive a free copy of my 'Breast Implants - Your Questions Answered' guide.

NOTES

NOTES

NOTES

NOTES

NOTES